ERECTILE DYSFUNCTION *Digest*

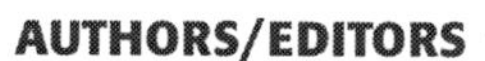

AUTHORS/EDITORS

ABHAY RANÉ, MS, FRCS (Urol)
Consultant Urological Surgeon, East Surrey Hospital, Redhill, Surrey, UK

MICHAEL FRASER, MB;ChB, FRCS (Urol)
Consultant Urological Surgeon, Stobhill Hospital, Glasgow, Scotland

CONTRIBUTORS

MONISH ARON, MCh, FRCS
Assistant Professor, All India Institute of Medical Sciences, New Delhi, India

PROKAR DASGUPTA, MD, FRCS
Consultant Urological Surgeon, Guy's Hospital, London, UK

ROBERTO MARIO SCARPA, MD
Professor of Urology, University of Turin, Orbassano, Italy

FOREWORD BY

DAVID M ALBALA, MD
Professor of Urology, Duke University Medical Center, Durham North Carolina, USA

Cover Design and Artwork by:

SMK Design

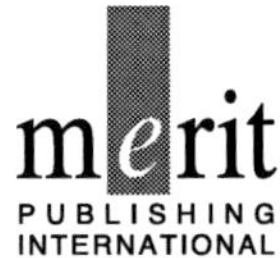

ERECTILE DYSFUNCTION
Digest

ISBN-13: 978 1 873413 69 2
ISBN-10: 1 873413 69 6

European Address:
50 Highpoint, Heath Road
Weybridge, Surrey KT13 8TP

Tel: 44(0)1932 844526
E-mail: merituk@aol.com

North American Address:
5840 Corporate Way, Suite 200
West Palm Beach, FL 33407

Tel: 561 697 1116
E-mail: meritpi@aol.com

Web: www.meritpublishing.com

A NOTE FROM DR. ABHAY RANE:

The aim of writing this book was to offer a concise, comprehensive and current overview of erectile dysfunction in a format that is easy-to-read, understand and convenient for quick reference.

I very much enjoyed working with a highly respected team of clinicians on this publication and hope that readers find it informative and useful.

CONTENTS

FOREWORD

The last decade has seen an enormous leap forward in the understanding of both the physiology of erection and the pathophysiologic processes behind erectile dysfunction (ED). Much research has been stimulated by the need to find effective, acceptable treatments for ED, and as such have been driven in part by the pharmaceutical industry, as well as by the medical profession. Prior to the introduction of Sildenafil, insertion of a penile prosthesis or self-injection was the only available option for a man with impotence. We now have an array of effective ED treatments, and stand on the threshold of an exciting era where men and their partners can opt to choose from a variety of options which best suit their individual lifestyles.

There do however, remain a group of men for whom current treatment is neither effective nor acceptable. We are therefore, continuing to strive to explore therapeutic avenues which may allow more patients to benefit and in the near future will see exciting ongoing research into the basic science of ED. Urologists will remain pivotal in this work.

The *Erectile Dysfunction Digest* is a practical and useful guide for clinicians dealing with problems related to erectile dysfunction. Dr. Abhay Rané, Dr. Michael Fraser and other contributors have developed a readable and practical guide for understanding erectile dysfunction and its treatments. The book, in an easy-to-use format, covers all the important areas, from epidemiology to pathophysiology and treatment of ED.

To complete the spectrum of andrology, Peyronie's disease is also covered, as this remains an important association with ED commonly encountered in urologic practice. Each of the chapters is well organized, practical, and readable. Practitioners at all levels will find this book useful, practical, and understandable.

David M. Albala, MD

INTRODUCTION

HISTORICAL ASPECTS

What is the difference between 'impotence' and 'erectile dysfunction'?

The term 'impotence' has traditionally been used to describe the inability to attain and maintain a satisfactory penile erection. However, since 1992 [1-2] this term has been replaced by 'erectile dysfunction' in order to distinguish the problem from other processes involved in male sexual dysfunction.

The word 'impotence' was derived from the Latin impotencia, which means lack of power. The term was first used in 1420 by Thomas Hoccleve [2] in his poem, 'De Regimine Principum' (The Government of Princes).

How did treatment of erectile dysfunction evolve into a science?

Much of the confusion about impotence through the ages arose as a direct result of lack of knowledge about the anatomy and physiology of penile erection. Leonardo da Vinci began interest in the anatomy of the penis and stated that erection was caused by engorgement of the penis with blood and not air, as was previously believed [11].

The first study of electronically induced erections was reported in 1863, when Eckhard showed an erection in canine models after stimulating the nervi erigentes. The first report of successful surgery for impotence was reported by Francesco Parona in 1873, when he sclerosed the varicose dorsal vein of the penis in a 30-year-old impotent man. Wooten in 1902, and Lydston in 1908 popularized the role of venous ligation for impotence, which was further developed by Hinman (1914). In 1936, Lowsley from New York reported a 60% success rate with plication of the ischiocavernosus and bulbocavernosus muscles [(2)].

The hormonal basis of erections first came to light in 1889 when Brown-Sequard, the famous French neurologist, at the age of 72, injected himself with an extract from the testicles of dogs and guinea pigs. He reported an increase in his mental and physical abilities, and by the end of 1889 over 12,000 physicians were administering this new 'Elixir of Life' [(12)].

The first three decades of the 20th century saw the emergence of vasal ligation [(13)], popularized as the 'Steinach operation', a method for rejuvenating sexual activity. Sigmund Freud and William Yeats are believed to have undergone this operation. From 1935, such rejuvenation operations lost their appeal because of the advent of organotherapy with xenotransplanted testicular tissue, or oral glandular extracts, beginning with the experiments of Serge Voronoff in 1918 [(2)].

In 1935, a group backed by a pharmaceutical company identified a new hormone in The Netherlands and the term 'testosterone' was coined for the first time (testo = testes, ster = sterol, one = ketone). In the same year, two groups artificially synthesized testosterone, thereby starting an industry that signaled the end of traditional 'organotherapy', and the use of these agents as oral aphrodisiacs continues to this day.

What about aphrodisiacs?

Aphrodisiacs take their name from Aphrodite, the Greek goddess of love. Mandrake, a member of the potato family, was mentioned as an aphrodisiac in the Old Testament (Genesis 30: 15) and Pliny, an ancient Greek in the First century AD, also noted it. The ancient Romans consumed the sexual organs of virile animals such as rabbits or dried tiger penises, which are still served today as soups in Taiwan and South Korea. The ancient Chinese drank the blood of deer and ate deer penises; even in these modern times, these are still considered a delicacy in some places.

Aristotle was the first person to mention cantharides as an aphrodisiac. The active ingredient, 'cantharidin', is extracted from the dried and powdered bodies of the blister beetle, also known as the Spanish Fly. Livia, wife of the Roman Emperor Tiberius, used to feed cantharides to other members of the Imperial family so that they might commit sexual indiscretions, thereby yielding material for blackmail [(14)].

Other animal based products that have been used as aphrodisiacs include snake blood, melted fat of camel hump, and a concoction of leeches. For various reasons, spicy foods and vanilla are also considered to have aphrodisiac properties [2]. Other foods have their aphrodisiac properties attributed to appearance and similarity to genital organs. The 'Doctrine of Signatures', from the Saxon times, states that 'every plant that is of use to man has been marked by God in a way that reveals its intended use'. Substances such as eggs, seeds and bulbs, oysters, avocado, cucumbers and carrots, ginseng, and the rhinoceros horn have all found use as aphrodisiacs [14]. Since Aphrodite was born at sea, many sea foods are thought to be powerful aphrodisiacs [2].

How did modern treatment methods of erectile dysfunction develop?

Prosthetic implants had their origins from plastic reconstructions of the penis after amputation [15]. Nicolai Borgoras [16] is credited with the first penile reconstruction (1936) adequate for micturition and sexual intercourse, using rib cartilage in a tube skin graft. The rib graft, however, was reabsorbed in a few months. After another failure of rib graft in 1948 from Bergman et al [17], the search began for an appropriate synthetic material. In 1952, Goodwin and Scott [18] used acrylic splints in five patients placed between the corpora cavernosa.

In 1966, Beheri [19] reported the use of polyethylene prostheses into each corpora in over 700 patients. In 1967, Pearman [20] reported the use of silastic intracavernosal implants, and the use of Hegar dilators to create the space. In 1973, Small et al [21] introduced the Small-Carrion semi-rigid paired prosthesis, which was later improved (Finney) to provide a hinge allowing penile flexion at the pubes [22]. In the same year, Scott et al introduced the inflatable implant controlled by subcutaneous scrotal pumps [2, 23].

Around the same time, in the mid 1970's, Geddings Osbon, a Pentecostal preacher who had founded a successful tire business, fashioned a prototype vacuum device from tire pumps [2]. In 1980, Ronald Virag [24], a French vascular surgeon, accidentally discovered the effects of intracavernosal injection of papaverine. In 1983, while presenting his work on intracavernosal phentolamine at the AUA meeting in Las Vegas, Giles Brindley, a 57-year-old Englishman, actually stepped in front of the podium and demonstrated his own erection from self-injection to the audience [12]!

In 1995, Alprostadil was marketed and it is now available for local injection or intraurethral delivery. Sildenafil has been studied since 1991 for its effect on anginal states, without much success. During trials in 1994, it was noted that this drug also increased blood flow to the penis and as a result improved erections. In 1998, the FDA gave approval for the use of sildenafil citrate as the first oral anti-impotence drug [2].

CHAPTER ONE

EPIDEMIOLOGY

How prevalent is ED?

The extent of ED has been estimated and reported in a number of population-based studies. Figures obtained in these studies vary significantly with the make-up of the group in question, in terms of factors including ethnicity, age group and associated co-morbidities. Therefore, any of the noted studies (and others) must be interpreted on their individual merits and cannot be used to necessarily inform on ED in other communities (Figures 1 & 2). Multi-national studies are few, but the MALES study gives important and interesting information on attitudes, prevalence and associated matters to men with ED.

Why should the prevalence of ED interest us?

It is clear from reported studies that ED represents a huge burden in terms of social impact of the condition and implicated treatment costs. This knowledge is vital to health economists in order that provision can be made at a national level to meet patients' needs. We also know however, that ED is associated with a wide variety of disease processes and as such we can infer that presentation with ED signifies the extent of other systemic problems.

Will the burden of ED change with time?

It has been extrapolated from existing data, that world-wide prevalence figures will increase dramatically in the period up to 2025. This assumption is based on the increase in longevity currently seen in most population groups and the association with age-related conditions of which ED and its clinical correlates may be included. Along with the expansion in available ED treatments and widened patient awareness, it seems likely that the socioeconomic burden of ED will rise dramatically.

STUDY	YEAR	POPULATION	PREVALENCE
Spector & Carey [2]	1990 1994,	Meta-analysis of English literature reported community studies	3-9%
Laumann et al [3-4]	1999	National Health and Social Life Survey	18-29 years, 7% 30-39 years, 9% 40-45 years, 11% 50-59 years, 18%
Feldman et al [5]	1994	Massachusetts Male Aging Study	ED-all degrees, 52% ED-minimal, 17.2% ED-moderate, 25.2% ED-complete, 9.6%

Figure 1. *ED in the United States*

STUDY	YEAR	POPULATION	PREVALENCE
Spector & Boyle [6]	1996	Britain, 109 patients	32%, difficulty obtaining erection 20%, difficulty maintaining erection
Malmsten et al [7]	1997	Sweden	7.6% overall rate of ED 1.5%, age 45 years 17.8%, age 80 years
Fugl-Meyer [8]	1999	Denmark, 1288 men	5%
Bejin [9]	1999	France	47%, overall rate of ED 7%, ED often
Chew et al [10]	2000	Australia, 1240 men	39.4% overall rate 9.6%, ED occasional 8.9%, ED often 18.6%, ED at all times

Figure 2. *ED in Europe and Australia*

CHAPTER TWO

PHYSIOLOGY & PATHOPHYSIOLOGY

How does penile erection occur?

The penile corporal bodies are the important structural elements in the erectile process. The substance of the corpora comprises a mass of smooth muscle and endothelial-lined vessels and spaces (lacunae), richly innervated with nerve endings. The encircling fibrous tunica albuginea provides structural integrity and has a secondary role in erection. The normally flaccid penis reflects a tonically contracted smooth muscle state, a position kept so by a sympathetic nervous input and the effect of inhibitory (or contractile) compounds derived from smooth muscle cells [(1)].

Sexual stimulation and arousal travels centrally via penile sensory nerves and parasympathetic fibers originating in the sacral segment of the spinal cord. Hypothalamic centers coordinate the various complex elements of the human sexual response and have a role in production of pro-erectile agents such as dopamine. The key however, to penile erection is the release of nitric oxide (NO) from cavernous nerve endings [(2)]. This neurotransmitter is pivotal in a cascade of cellular events, which result in smooth muscle relaxation and vasodilatation of the helicine arteries. Subsequently, this leads to increased blood flow and penile lacunar expansion. Compression of small veins in the tunica prevents blood flow out of the penis and along with NO derived from the endothelium, maintains erection.

How is the penis maintained in its normal flaccid state?

In the non-erect penis, the corporal smooth muscle exists in a contracted state. This represents the effect of overriding sympathetic nervous control in the absence of sexual stimulation but additional release of pro-contractile substances also plays an important role. Endothelial cells are known to release endothelin-1 and prostaglandin F2a, which act as vasoconstrictors to limit blood flow into the penis. Other substances, such as angiotensin II and neuropeptide Y, may also play a contributory role.

What is erectile dysfunction?

Erectile dysfunction (ED) is defined as "the consistent or recurrent inability to attain and/or maintain penile erection sufficient for sexual performance"

What is the etiology of erectile dysfunction?

As erection is primarily a vascular event, any process affecting blood flow into the penis may result in ED. A number of identified risk factors are outlined below. In general terms, the severity of ED may vary with the number of risk factors in any individual.

Risk Factors:

- Ageing
- Diabetes
- Hypertension
- Dyslipidemia
- Smoking

All the above are now established as common etiological factors in both atherosclerotic cardiovascular disease and ED, but it is also clear that ageing and diabetes have direct effects on the cellular function. Ageing has been shown to be associated with down regulation of NO-sensitive pathways and in diabetes there is demonstrable evidence of impaired relaxation of smooth muscle in response to NO.

More recent studies also have shown elevated levels of vasoconstrictor substances (Endothelin-1 and Angiotensin Converting Enzyme) with reduction of NO and cGMP in the blood of ED patients of various etiologies. These suggest that primary endothelial cell dysfunction may play a significant role in ED.

What is the metabolic syndrome?

The term 'metabolic syndrome' is used to define a cluster or profile of adverse clinical components, which may be viewed as risk factors for cardiovascular disease. Different bodies, including the WHO, identify slightly different components to this syndrome (listed below), but these share common endpoints in terms of adverse CVS events including ED.

Components of the metabolic syndrome:

- Abdominal obesity
- Atherogenic dyslipidemia
- Raised blood pressure
- Insulin resistance +/_ glucose intolerance
- Proinflammatory state
- Prothrombotic state

What are other conditions associated with ED?

Apart from the common risk profile with cardiovascular disease, a number of conditions or disease processes are strongly associated with ED and are listed below. For some, the link is clear if one remembers the normal erectile processes and hence possible areas where these may be interfered. In other cases, the association with lower urinary tract symptoms, for instance, the mechanism whereby erectile function is disrupted is less clear.

Neural

Disorders of both central or peripheral nerve pathways involved in erection may result in ED. Commonly quoted CNS associations are Parkinson's disease (60%), multiple sclerosis (70%), stroke (30%), dementia (Alzheimer's) and major depressive illness. Less commonly, brain tumors or trauma may be implicated. However, spinal cord lesions are an important cause of ED in all age groups. Lesions of the sacral cord are associated with ED in up to 80% whereas a figure nearer 10% is seen in those with suprasacral lesions.

Endocrine

Diabetes mellitus is the major contributor to ED. Diabetes not only has a causative role in vasculopathy associated with ED, but it may also affect neural control of erection (peripheral somatic or autonomic) and be related to local degenerative changes in corporal smooth muscle and tunica. Raised plasma glucose levels and advanced glycation end products (AGEs) may also be important in the development of cellular dysfunction.

Other endocrine abnormalities are certainly less frequent factors in etiology, but hypogonadism must always be considered as a potentially reversible factor. The precise role of androgen deficiency clinically (particularly in the ageing male) remains controversial to an extent, but androgens have been demonstrated to have a role in smooth muscle function in the penis. Hyperprolactinemia is rare, but may accompany other conditions such as diabetes and renal or liver failure.

Local factors

We have already stated that diabetes may have an effect on cellular/tunical function. Other conditions such as Peyronie's disease and atherosclerosis may also result in veno-occlusive dysfunction ("venous leak"). Direct interference with neural innervation of the penis may be caused by various forms of pelvic surgery (e.g. radical prostatectomy, proctocolectomy) or by radiation therapy.

CHAPTER THREE

INVESTIGATION AND EVALUATION

How should the ED patient be evaluated?

It is important to have the patient's salient history. Specific points to be included are:

- **Diseases:** chronic renal failure, diabetes mellitus, chronic liver failure, chronic alcoholism, and neurologic disease.
- **Atherosclerosis risk factors:** cigarette smoking, older age, diabetes mellitus, obesity, hypertension, hyperlipidemia.
- **Surgery:** radical prostatectomy, radical cystectomy, proctocolectomy, aorto-iliac arterial surgery, aortic aneurysm repair, any pituitary, penile, pelvic, urethral, or prostatic surgery.
- **Trauma:** pelvic fracture, penile fracture, blunt perineal/pelvic/penile trauma, back or spinal injury.
- **Other factors:** depression or other psychiatric disorder, priapism, pelvic radiation, alcohol abuse.

- **Medications:** antihypertensives (especially beta-blockers, thiazides, clonidine, methyldopa), anticholinergics, antidepressants and antipsychotics (especially tricyclic antidepressants, MAO inhibitors, lithium, and phenothiazines).

- **Sexual history:** onset and duration of ED, maximum rigidity, sustaining capability, capable of penetrative intercourse or not, nocturnal penile tumescence, erections with masturbation, last successful intercourse, frequency of intercourse currently and one year prior to the onset of the problem, libido, recent psychological stress, ejaculatory dysfunction, orgasmic dysfunction, penile curvature.

Clinical Examination

The extent of clinical examination of the ED patient remains controversial. Certainly, genital inspection and palpation for conditions such as Peyronie's disease would seem essential as would assessment of the peripheral vasculature. Neurological examination and digital rectal examination are not mandatory, though may be influenced by particular patient or investigative factors.

What is the IIEF?

The International Index of Erectile Function (IIEF) is a written questionnaire used to facilitate and standardize communication when discussing sexual dysfunction. The core element (EF domain) is a five-item questionnaire to which a score of 1 to 5 is returned for each question, where 1 is the least and 5 is the most functional response. ED severity is classified into five categories based on the IIEF-5: Severe (5 to 7), Moderate (8-11), Mild to moderate (12 to 16), Mild (17 to 21), No ED (22 to 25).

The most widely used role of the IIEF is in reporting of clinical trial data, where it is used as a baseline marker and end of study assessment of ED severity. In this situation, it is commonly reported alongside patient responses to the Sexual Encounter Profile questions (SEP 2 & SEP3), which relate to ability to penetrate (SEP2) and to complete intercourse (SEP3).

What tests are indicated in ED patients?

It must be realized that a complete series of diagnostic tests may provide very little added value, and may be tailored according to the wishes of the patient and the goals of therapy

WHO guidelines recommend a fasting serum glucose and lipid profile as the only mandatory first line invasive tests, with subsequent investigation tailored to individual circumstances. Many clinicians now use blood for testosterone estimation (a morning sample), as this may be useful information for those who do not respond to first line therapy. However, the precise contribution of androgen deficiency to both broad populations and individuals remains unclear in many respects.

Can you describe the available tests in detail?

- **Penile duplex ultrasonography and Doppler analysis:** Uses 5-10 Hz transducers to image the penis 5-10 minutes after intracavernous injection of an erectogenic medication. This test measures the arterial flow, which is examined in each of the cavernous arteries.

- **Cavernous artery peak systolic velocity (PSV):** normal > 30 cm/s, severe arterial insufficiency < 25 cm/s. The sum of right and left cavernous artery PSV should be >50-60 cm/s to rule out arteriogenic ED. Peak velocity should be measured with the probe-vessel doppler angle at 60°.

- **Cavernous artery diameter:** normal flaccid diameter = 0.3-0.4 mm, normal erect diameter = 0.7-1.2 mm. Arteriogenic insufficiency is suspected if erect cavernous artery diameter is <0.7 mm.

- **Cavernous artery end diastolic velocity (EDV):** normal ≤3 cm/s. With isolated veno-occlusive disease, PSV is normal and EDV >3 cm/s.

When would you use combined intracavernous injection and stimulation?

This is used as an initial test to evaluate the functional status of the erectile mechanism. The patient undergoes intracavernous injection and stimulates himself to achieve erection; the optimal intracavernosal medication and its dosage have not been established. Furthermore, standard criteria of what constitutes a normal test have not been established. A good erection rules out venous insufficiency, but does NOT rule out arterial insufficiency. A poor response can result from: inadequate intracavernosal dosing or administration, venous insufficiency, arterial insufficiency, or extreme anxiety.

What is cavernosometry ?

This is the most sensitive test to detect veno-occlusive dysfunction. Intracavernosal pressures are measured during an intracavernous injection with an erectogenic drug such as papaverine or alprostadil. In addition, a heparinized saline infusion into the corpora is used to maintain the intracavernosal pressure at a selected value.

Flow to maintain:

If veno-occlusive dysfunction is present, then blood will flow out of the corpora, the intracavernosal pressure will fall, and the heparinised saline infusion rate will have to be increased in order to maintain the intracavernosal pressure. The flow of saline into the corpora to maintain intracavernosal pressure is called the "flow to maintain." Veno-occlusive dysfunction is considered to be present when the flow to maintain is > 3 ml/minute.

Intracavernosal pressure decay:

The cavernosal pressure is set at 150 mm Hg and the heparinized saline infusion is then turned off. If the intracavernosal pressure declines by 45 mm Hg or more in 30 seconds, this suggests veno-occlusive dysfunction.

Cavernosography:

This is usually performed at the same time as cavernosometry. After intracavernosal pharmacotherapy, radiographic contrast is infused instead of saline to maintain flow and both anteroposterior and oblique images are obtained. This test is used to visualize the location of the venous leak.

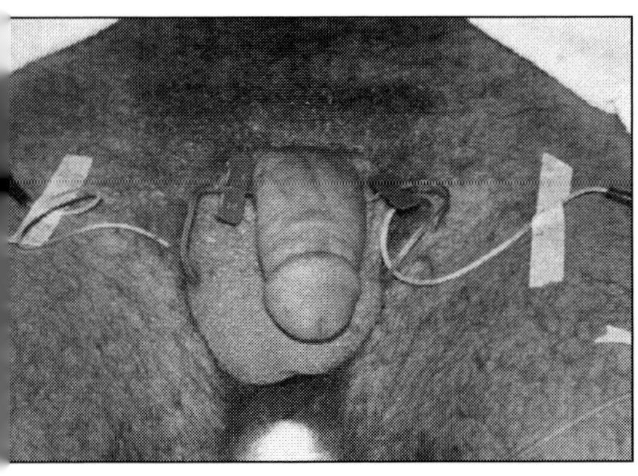

Interpretation:

with normal veno-occlusive function, no venous drainage from the corpora is seen on cavernosography (i.e. only the corpora are visualized during erection)

Cavernosography. *Courtesy of Mr Suks Minhas The Institute of Urology, London*

What are Nocturnal Penile Tumescence and Rigidity (NPTR)?

These relate to methods for detecting erections ± degree of rigidity during REM sleep. These methods include Rigiscan observation, strain gauges, and plethysmography (uses a blood pressure cuff type device to approximate intracavernous pressure).

Measuring NPTR may help distinguish psychogenic erectile dysfunction from organic causes. However, NPTR must be interpreted with great caution. NPTR can be confounded by many non-psychogenic factors, including sleep disturbances, dream content, certain neurologic conditions, and medications.. Erections during sleep cannot always be equated with erections during sexual activity.

NPTR is neither sensitive nor specific enough to use as a single diagnostic evaluation and it is usually not a routine part of the ED work up. NPTR is mainly indicated when psychogenic ED is suspected or in medico-legal cases to ascertain ability of the individual to penetrate. The NPTR should take place for at least two nights. The presence of an erectile event of at least 70 % rigidity recorded on the tip of the penis, lasting for 10 minutes or more, should be considered as indicative of a functional erectile mechanism

What is internal pudendal arteriography and when is it indicated?

This is the gold standard for demonstrating arterial insufficiency and is only indicated in young men with suspected arterial insufficiencies that are candidates for revascularization procedures.

What is the Cavernous Arterial Systolic Occlusion Pressure (CASOP)?

After intracavernosal pharmacotherapy, this test uses a blood pressure cuff-like system to determine at what pressure the cavernous artery flow becomes detectable. Arteriogenic ED is probably present when the following equation is true: (Brachial systolic pressure > CASOP +35 mm Hg). CASOP is sometimes performed in conjunction with cavernosometry.

Other tests include:

- Penile brachial index (PBI): measured in the flaccid state. PBI $\leq$ 0.7 implies arteriogenic ED.
- Psychological testing.
- Radioisotope penography (has been used to demonstrate veno-occlusive dysfunction).

Interpretation: What are the indicators of Arteriogenic ED?

Test results should show:

- Cavernous artery PSV < 25 cm/s or sum of right and left cavernous artery PSV < 50 cm/s.
- Brachial systolic arterial pressure > CASOP +35 mm Hg.
- Occlusive lesion identified on internal pudendal arteriography.
- Dilation of cavernosal artery to < 0.7 mm.
- PBI ≤ 0.7.

What are the indicators of Veno-occlusive ED?

Test results should show:

- Flow to maintain > 3 ml/minute.
- Intracavernosal pressure decay by 45 mm Hg or more in 30 seconds.
- Venous leak seen on cavernosography.
- Cavernous artery EDV >3 cm/s.

What are the indicators of Psychogenic ED?

Test results should show:

- Rigid erections with NPTR.
- Good erection with combined intracavernosal injection and stimulation test.
- Normal arterial and veno-occlusive function on other tests.

Practical Assessment of the patient with ED

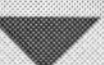

Comprehensive medical and psychological history from patient and partner

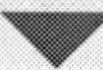

International Index for Erectile Function (IIEF)

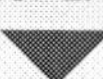

Focused physical examination genitourinary, endocrine, vascular, neurologic

Mandatory

Blood glucose

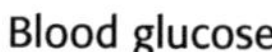

Optional

PSA, Testosterone, Prolactin Lipids

Specific testing

- In primary ED when beside pychogenic disorders, organic disease should be excluded
- Young patients with pelvic or perineal trauma
- Patients who could potentially benefit from vascular surgery.

- Nocturnal penile tumescence and rigidity (Rigiscan for at least two nights)
- Intracavernosal injection test (IIT)
- Duplex ultrasound (DU) of penis if IIT inconclusive
- Arteriography or cavernosometry if DU inconclusive
- Bulbocavernosal reflex latency
- Nerve conduction studies
- Endocrinological evaluation by endocrinologist
- Psychodiagnostic evaluation by psychiatrist.

CHAPTER FOUR

TREATMENT OPTIONS

What are the treatment options for Erectile Dysfunction?

Although penile prostheses remain one of the most effective treatments of all types of ED, the current recommendations focus on a stepladder approach to the management of the patient with ED. The stepladder (see algorithm in chapter 8), progresses from non-invasive drug therapy to minimally invasive injection therapy or vacuum devices to more invasive prosthetic surgery.

The introduction of sildenafil in the late 1990's revolutionized the drug treatment of ED making it the first line of therapy against this disorder. Although over the years, it has become clear there is no 'magic bullet' for all patients with ED, the significant benefits experienced by a large number of patients with varied etiologies has spurred scientists to initiate the search for better oral drugs for this malady. Apart from these goal-directed specific therapies, various non-specific methods that include dietary and lifestyle alterations and psychosexual counseling are also of great importance, and the patient needs to be made aware of all available modalities of treatment, their benefits and side-effects, in order to make an informed decision.

General recommendations

- Stop smoking – Smoking increases the risk of ED, by its effects on the vasculature, and also as a result of the side effects of the drugs used to treat effects of cardiovascular disease

- Weight loss (if the patient is obese)

- Reduce alcohol intake – alcohol in small amounts improves erection and sexual desire; however large amounts can cause central sedation, decreased libido, and transient ED. Chronic alcoholism may result in liver dysfunction, decreased testosterone and increased estrogen levels, and alcoholic polyneuropathy, which may also affect penile nerves

- If the patient takes prescription medication that may contribute to ED, conduct a thorough medicines review

- Ensure good control of diabetes mellitus – ED has been estimated to occur in 35% to 75% of men with diabetes mellitus. Diabetes may cause ED through its effect on the CNS and peripheral nerve function, psychological issues, androgen production, vascular angiopathy, and endothelial and smooth muscle function.

Psychogenic ED

Psychogenic factors are involved either alone or in combination with organic causes in a substantial number of cases of erectile dysfunction. Epidemiologic studies have implicated a depressed mood, loss of self-esteem, and other psychosocial stresses in the etiology of erectile dysfunction. However, the diagnosis of psychogenic ED must remain one of exclusion, in order to avoid overlooking treatable organic causes.

Traditional treatment approaches have included anxiety reduction and desensitization procedures, cognitive-behavioral interventions, guided sexual stimulation techniques, and couples or relationship counseling. Minimally invasive and highly effective therapies such as sildenafil citrate, vacuum constriction device, or ICI may sometimes be better than a prolonged course of psychosexual therapy with its attendant compliance issues. However, in some cases psychosexual therapy should be the first intervention, particularly if it can eliminate the specific underlying cause.

- Suggest counseling

- Any of the therapies for assisted erection may be tried (see chapter 7) Start with the least invasive therapies, i.e., lifestyle alterations and drugs. Sometimes these may be used temporarily until the psychogenic cause has been overcome.

Neurogenic or mixed ED

Neurogenic ED can be defined as inability to sustain or maintain a penile erection due to a neurologic impairment or dysfunction. Because erection is a neurovascular event, any disease, or dysfunction affecting the brain, spinal cord, cavernous and pudendal nerves, or receptors in the terminal arterioles and cavernous smooth muscle can induce dysfunction. Effect of a neurologic deficit on penile erections is complex, and, with a few exceptions, neurological testing rarely changes management. There is no reliable test to assess neurotransmitter release, which leaves a significant gap in the current assessment of neurological function associated with erection.

Any of the therapies for assisted erection may be tried (start with the least invasive therapies). Men with neurogenic impotence respond more dramatically to pharmacological erection therapies; therefore, they should be started at lower doses compared to men with other types of erectile dysfunction.

In what way does Renal Failure cause ED?

Chronic renal failure has frequently been associated with diminished erectile function, impaired libido, and sub-fertility. The mechanism is probably multi-factorial; depressed testosterone and elevation of prolactin levels, diabetes mellitus, vascular insufficiency, multiple medications, autonomic and somatic neuropathy, and psychological stress.

Men with significant renal failure may have erectile dysfunction. Those with end stage renal disease may find resolution of the ED after a renal transplant. In patients who are candidates for kidney transplant, therefore, a penile prosthesis is avoided, and less invasive treatment options are persevered with.

Hormonal therapy

Androgens affect the growth and development of the male reproductive tract and secondary sexual characteristics.

Testosterone

(a) enhances sexual interest
(b) increases frequency of sexual acts
(c) increases the frequency of nocturnal erections.

Any dysfunction of the hypothalamic-pituitary axis can result in hypogonadism, with a resultant decrease in testosterone production. Aging men may have hypogonadism. Serum testosterone levels decrease as age increases because the number of Leydig cells fall. Therefore, in patients with documented hypogonadism and ED, it appears appropriate to initiate androgen therapy. Patients with thyroid, adrenal, pituitary, or hypothalamic dysfunction should, however, be referred to an endocrinologist for management.

Low testosterone

Contraindications to testosterone replacement: known or suspected prostate or male breast cancer, significant risk for prostate cancer, severe liver dysfunction, severe polycythemia, congestive heart failure, severe sleep apnea (relative contraindications include hyperlipidemia, hypercholesterolemia, mild polycythemia, mild sleep apnea)

Testosterone replacement may:

- Cause hepatic problems (hepatitis, hepatic neoplasms)
- Cause polycythemia and hypercholesterolemia
- Cause fluid retention, pulmonary edema, and congestive heart failure in patients with cardiac, renal, or hepatic disease
- May increase anticoagulant levels and increase the risk of bleeding
- May worsen sleep apnea
- Cause hypoglycemia in diabetics taking insulin. When diabetics are started on testosterone, blood sugar should be monitored closely and insulin should be adjusted accordingly.

Baseline blood tests should be drawn prior to therapy and monitored periodically (consider every six months). These tests include: hemoglobin, hematocrit, liver function tests, prostate specific antigen, and cholesterol HDL (also PT/PTT for patients on anticoagulant therapy). A digital rectal examination to assess the prostate should be performed before treatment and at least every six months.

Testosterone replacement in men with normal pre-treatment PSA does not alter PSA or PSA velocity beyond established norms; therefore, any abnormality in PSA during therapy should not be attributed to testosterone replacement.

Which forms of testosterone supplementation are available?

- **Intramuscular:** Testosterone enanthate or testosterone cypionate 200-300 mg IM every two to three weeks (adjust dose and frequency based on testosterone levels). Testosterone levels should reach normal by one week. This route of administration results in high peak and low trough testosterone levels; this therefore does not replicate normal circadian levels.

- **Transdermal:** This route of administration results in more stable testosterone levels without high peaks and low troughs.

Androgen patch, 2.5 to 7.5 mg in a 24- hour period. Patches come in 2.5 and 5 mg. Starting dose is 5 mg q 24 hours (adjust dose based on testosterone levels, which peak 8-12 hours later). Patients are advised not to apply to bony prominences, scrotum, or areas subject to prolonged pressure, and to change the application area daily. Side effects may include itching, skin irritation, and allergic contact dermatitis.

Androgen gel, 5 to 10 g sachet in a 24-hour period. Each sachet contains 50 mg testosterone in 5 g colorless gel. Start with 5 g sachet, and adjust dose in 2.5 g aliquots to a maximum of 10 g in a 24-hour period. Patients are advised not to apply to bony prominences, scrotum, or areas subject to prolonged pressure, and to change the application area daily. Side effects may include itching, skin irritation, and allergic contact dermatitis.

- **Oral:** Oral testosterone is largely rendered metabolically inactive during first-pass circulation through liver and is associated with a high rate of hepatotoxic side effects. It is not a favored route of testosterone administration.

Which therapies are available for assisted erections?

The therapies available for assisted erections are:

- Vacuum devices
- Intraurethral injections: prostaglandins
- Drugs: PDE5 inhibitors, yohimbine, apomorphine
- Intracavernosal injections: papaverine, prostaglandins, alpha-blockers

General considerations:

These therapies should not be used in men whom sexual activity is inadvisable or contraindicated. All patients who use intracavernosal pharmacotherapy are at risk for priapism. The patients must be counseled about the risk of priapism and are advised to seek medical attention promptly if priapism occurs. The lowest possible dose to achieve erection should be used to minimize the risk of priapism and other side effects. None of these therapies should be used in patients with penile tumors until the tumor has been treated.

What is a vacuum erection device (VED)?

A cylinder is placed over the penis and a vacuum pump draws blood into the penis. An occlusive band is placed around the base of the penis to maintain the erection.

Contraindications:

- any predisposition to priapism,
- significant angulation or fibrosis of the penis
- penile implant
- bleeding disorder or anticoagulation

Maximum duration of use: 20-30 minutes. Maximum frequency of use: wait at least one hour after removing the occlusive band before using the VED again

What is a venous constriction band?

This is a circular band that fits around the base of the penis. It can be used alone or in combination with other therapies for assisted erections (except penile prostheses). The least constrictive tension that will maintain an erection is utilized for no longer than 20 minutes.

Intraurethral

The drug is injected intraurethrally through the external urethral meatus and is transferred from the urethra to the corpus spongiosum and then to the corpus cavernosum through venous channels.

MUSE® (**M**edical **U**rethral **S**ystem for **E**rection) is based on the discovery that the urethra (the tube passing from the bladder to the tip of the penis through which urine is passed and semen ejaculated) can absorb certain medications, which can then pass into the surrounding erectile tissue creating an erection.

Alprostadil (prostaglandin E1) is the active ingredient in MUSE. Alprostadil relaxes the muscles in the erectile tissue of the penis allowing increased blood flow, the basis of a normal erection. It acts through a membrane receptor that activates adenylate cyclase, therefore it increases levels of intracellular cyclic AMP. It also inhibits platelet aggregation. In MUSE, alprostadil is formulated as a small pellet, which is supplied in a specially designed applicator in which each is individually wrapped. The applicator's narrow stem can be introduced easily into the urethra and after inserting the applicator, the pellet is released by depressing a button.

Immediately prior to insertion of MUSE, it is recommended that the patient urinates and then gently shakes the penis several times to remove excess urine. A moist urethra makes administration of MUSE easier and facilitates the absorption of alprostadil.

Erection begins 5-20 minutes after administration.

Contraindications:

- any predisposition to priapism,
- significant angulation or fibrosis of the penis,
- penile implant
- distal urethral stricture
- urethritis

Side effects:

- Pain/burning in the penis or urethra
- urethral bleeding
- priapism
- hypotension
- headache
- dizziness.

Dose:

- Maximum Dose = 1000 mcg
- Maximum dosing frequency = two times per 24 hours. An erection should completely detumesce before another dose is administered.

CHAPTER FIVE

PHOSPHODIESTERASE INHIBITORS

What are phosphodiesterase inhibitors?

The phosphodiesterase inhibitors, or more specifically, phosphodiesterase type 5 inhibitors (PDE5), are a class of agent with a specific action upon cyclic nucleotide signaling. This signaling system is closely regulated by the levels of the nucleotides cAMP and cGMP, which in turn are determined by synthesis of adenylate or guanylate cyclase enzymes, and by inactivation by the PDE systems. PDEs are widespread throughout biological systems and are divided into 11 families. PDE5 has the widest tissue distribution and is also the prime PDE involved in erectile physiology.

What are the currently available PDE5s?

Sildenafil

Sildenafil inhibits type 5 cGMP phosphodiesterase, which is primarily located in the cavernosal smooth muscle. Sildenafil is significantly better than placebo at achieving successful sexual intercourse and has been proven to have an excellent safety profile over the past five years. It does not generate an erection; therefore, stimulation must occur to generate an erection.

Contraindications
This drug is contraindicated in patients taking nitrates (sildenafil potentiates the effects of these medications, which may cause life threatening hypotension)

Side effects
Include (most to least common): headache, flushing, dyspepsia, nasal congestion, abnormal vision (abnormal color tinge, increased sensitivity to light, blurred vision), diarrhea, dizziness, rash.

Dose:
- Maximum dose = 100 mg
- Maximum dosing frequency = once per day
- Initial dose: Sildenafil 50 mg po one hour before sexual activity.

In patients taking cytochrome P450 3A4 inhibitors (e.g. erythromycin, ketoconazole, etc.), age >65, liver impairment, or severe renal impairment (creatinine clearance < 30 ml/min), the initial dose is sildenafil 25 mg po one hour before sexual activity. Titrate dose from 25 to 100 mg based on erectile response and side effects.

Vardenafil
Vardenafil is a novel inhibitor of phosphodiesterase type 5. It is significantly better than placebo at achieving successful sexual intercourse. This drug has been shown to be effective in a group of patients who were not responsive to sildenafil.

Contraindications

For patients taking nitrates; men for whom sexual activity is inadvisable (e.g. very severe cardiovascular disorders); severe hepatic impairment; end stage renal disease requiring dialysis; hypotension; recent stroke or myocardial ischemia; unstable angina; and known hereditary retinal degenerative disorders.

Side effects

Include flushing, headache, dyspepsia, nausea, dizziness, rhinitis, hypertension, photosensitivity reaction, abnormal vision, hypertonia, hypotension, syncope, and erectile disturbance.

Dose:

- Maximum dose = 20 mg
- Maximum dosing frequency = once per day
- Initial dose: 10 mg orally 25 to 60 minutes before sexual activity. Based on efficacy and tolerability the dose may be increased to 20 mg or decreased to 5mg.

This medication may be taken with or without food; however, onset may be delayed if taken with a high fat meal.

Tadalafil

Tadalafil is a novel inhibitor of phosphodiesterase type 5. It is significantly better than placebo at achieving successful sexual intercourse. It has a maximum serum peak of 2.0 h and a long half-life of 17.5 h that is associated with erectogenic potential lasting for 24 h. This may allow patients to engage in sexual activity more than once after a single administration.

Contraindications

Include patients taking nitrates; men for whom sexual activity is inadvisable (e.g. very severe cardiovascular disorders); severe hepatic impairment; end stage renal disease requiring dialysis; hypotension; recent stroke or myocardial ischemia; unstable angina; and known hereditary retinal degenerative disorders.

Side effects

Include flushing, headache, dyspepsia, nausea, dizziness, rhinitis, conjunctival hyperemia, back pain, and myalgia.

Dose:

- Maximum dose = 20 mg
- Maximum dosing frequency = once per day
- Initial dose: 10 mg orally 30 minutes to 12 h before sexual activity. Based on efficacy and tolerability the dose may be increased to 20 mg. This medication may be taken with or without food; however, onset may be delayed if taken with a high fat meal.

Which is the "best" PDE5 inhibitor?

There is no answer to this question. There have been no direct head-to-head studies between any of the drugs and there may never be any comparisons. Some would suggest that design of such a study would prove almost impossible to determine efficacy of one drug over another, particularly with the rather subjective, personalized endpoints used in most ED drug trials.

Similarly, patient groups and methods vary significantly between published studies of all three drugs, such that direct comparisons are not possible. It can be said however, that despite pharmacokinetic differences, this class of drug shares similar effects and outcomes.

Sildenafil, vardenafil and tadalafil have all been shown in randomized controlled trials (RCTs) to be effective in broad populations of men with varying ED etiologies. Early studies centered on effects on nocturnal penile tumescence as proof of principle. All three PDE5s demonstrated improvements in NPT when compared to placebo.

Phase III studies of similar design, have all shown significant improvements in IIEF from baseline compared to placebo. Currently, studies are reporting on patient preference data. This area remains difficult to interpret, with variable inclusion and design criteria. Additionally, the inherent personal complexities of the human sexual response make this an area where the reader should exert caution in interpretation of data.

What is "difficult-to-treat" ED?

The presence of certain risk factors appears to make the degree of ED more severe. It has long been appreciated that accumulation of several adverse cardiovascular stigmata contributes to a greater ED severity, but we can now add the presence of diabetes to this group. Diabetic patients will in general develop ED earlier in life and to a greater severity than non-diabetic age-matched counterparts.

To this difficult-to-treat group should also be included men who have undergone radical prostatectomy or radiation therapy for prostate cancer. Intact penile innervation is vital for normal erection to occur, and both surgical and radiation-induced injury may affect this mechanism. It should also be remembered that intact penile nerves are postulated to be required for PDE5s to exert their action.

How do the PDE5s fare in these "difficult-to-treat" groups?

Diabetes

In the published sildenafil diabetes study, 56% of men reported improved erections compared to 10% on placebo ($p<0.001$) and more than 60% had at least one successful intercourse attempt during the 12 weeks of the study. Similarly, vardenafil improved erectile function (in terms of IIEF score) over placebo in a dose-response relationship using 10 and 20mg doses. In a trial of the same design using tadalafil, EF domain scores showed changes from baseline of 0.1 with placebo but 6.4 with 10mg ($p<0.001$ versus placebo) and 7.3 for 20mg tadalafil ($p<0.001$ versus placebo). It should be noted that an increase of 4 in the EF domain score is deemed to be clinically significant in these studies.

Prostatectomy

In an open-label study of sildenafil after radical prostatectomy (RP), 53% of men reported improved erections with either the 50 or 100mg dose. A three year follow-up study in a cohort of post-prostatectomy patients in whom an approximately 50% response at one year was observed, showed that the majority of these (72%) who showed an initial response were still effectively managed by sildenafil at three years.

A phase III study using vardenafil showed improved EF domain scores with a response rate using the GAQ (secondary endpoint) of approximately 70% in the group using the 20mg dose. In tadalafil studies, similar findings were observed with 62% of men taking 20mg showing improvement in a study of approximately 300 men with ED seen 12-48 months after RP.

For all the PDE5 studies in patients post-RP, erectile function is strongly related to the degree of nerve-sparing during the surgery itself, and to the patient's pre-operative erectile status. Some data is available on the potential for restoration of post-prostatectomy erections by early or prophylactic treatment with both injection and PDE5 therapy, but this requires further work.

CHAPTER SIX

OTHER PHARMACOLOGIC AGENTS

In the PDE5 era, what other drugs still have a role in ED?

Not all men with ED have a satisfactory response to PDE5 inhibitors, and a further proportion have direct contraindications to their usage (e.g. nitrate medication). For these patients, alternative oral agents are currently disappointing in their efficacy and realistically have little place in modern ED management. We will discuss both apomorphine and yohimbine in the following section.

Apomorphine

This is a centrally acting dopamine agonist, which works by activating the dopamine receptors in the para-ventricular nucleus within the hypothalamus. Subsequently, this causes direct neural erectile stimulation.

Side effects

Nausea, vomiting, yawning, sweating

Contraindications

Moderate heart failure and unstable angina

Dose

- 2 mg sublingually, increased cautiously to 3 mg.
- Maximum daily dose 2 mg 8 hourly.

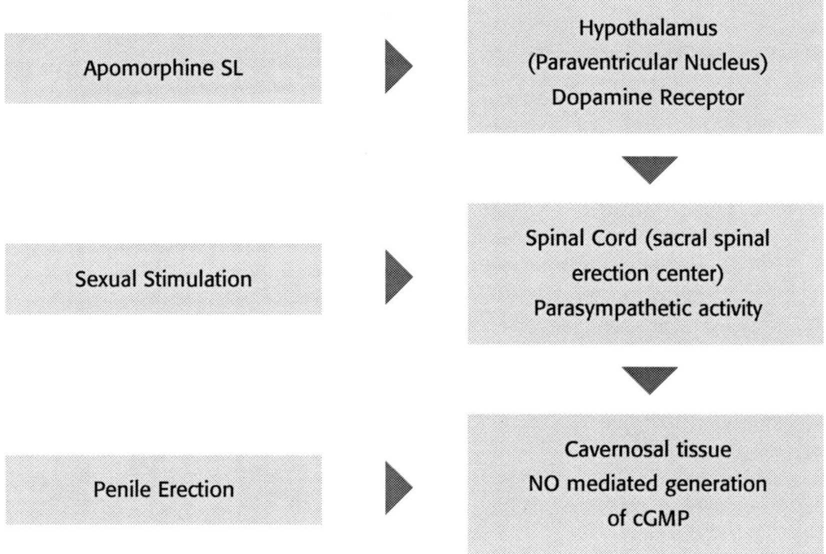

Yohimbine

This agent blocks presynaptic alpha-2 adrenergic receptors and therefore it tends to increase parasympathetic and decrease sympathetic activity. It is not significantly better than placebo in patients with organic ED. It may be of some benefit in patients with psychogenic ED.

Contraindications
Include renal insufficiency, cardiac dysfunction or arrhythmia, peptic ulcer disease, hypertension, concomitant use with other mood modifying drugs.

Side effects
Anxiety, irritability, anti-diuresis, increased blood pressure, increased heart rate, tremor, sweating, nausea, vomiting, dizziness, headache.

Dose
5.4 mg tablet orally three times daily. If side effects are troublesome, the dose is halved. It may take several weeks until an effect is observed.

Can you describe the role for intracavernosal injection therapy?

Direct intracavernosal injection of vasoactive agents generally provide rapid, reliable penile erections in all but the most severe cases of arterial insufficiency. While effective, this approach to treatment is less acceptable to patients than oral drugs, and discontinuation of use due to lack of tolerability is a major issue. In the U.K., prostaglandin E1 (Alprostadil) is most widely used, but papaverine, sodium nitroprusside and various combinations may be seen in other practices.

Alprostadil

Act through a membrane receptor that activates adenylate cyclase; therefore, it increases levels of intracellular cyclic AMP. Erection begins 5-20 minutes after injection.

Contraindications:

- any predisposition to priapism
- significant angulation or fibrosis of the penis
- penile implant

Side effects:

- penile pain/burning (in up to 37%),
- priapism,
- penile fibrosis (up to 8%),
- hypotension
- headache

Dose:

- Maximum dose = 60 mcg
- Maximum dosing frequency = 3 times per week with at least 24-hours between each dose.
- Initial dosing should be titrated carefully. In patients with neurogenic impotence start with alprostadil 1.25 mcg intracavernous injection. If response is insufficient, increase the dose in increments

of 1.25 mcg. In patients with mixed or non-neurogenic impotence start with alprostadil 2.5 mcg intracavernous injection. If response is insufficient, increase the dose in increments of 5 mcg.

Papaverine

This drug inhibits phosphodiesterase, thereby preventing the degradation of cAMP.

Contraindications

Patients with any predisposition to priapism, significant angulation or fibrosis of the penis, or a penile implant.

Side effects

Include: priapism, fibrosis of erectile tissue.

Dose (titration to the appropriate dose should be carefully supervised by a physician):

- Initial dose: In patients with neurogenic impotence start with papaverine 3 mg intracavernous injection.
- In patients with mixed or non-neurogenic impotence start with papaverine 5-10 mg intracavernous injection; if response is insufficient, increase the dose in small increments.
- Maximum dosing frequency should probably be 3 times per week with at least 24 hours between each dose.

CHAPTER SEVEN

SURGERY

What are the indications for insertion of a penile prosthesis?

When corpora cavernosal tissue is no longer functional because of replacement by a certain amount of fibrous tissue, the only solution for ED may be the implantation of a penile prosthesis. In addition, patients who do not respond adequately to, or do not tolerate the previously mentioned therapies for assisted erection, may also be candidates for a penile prosthesis. Simply stated, a penile prosthesis is a mechanical device that is implanted within the corpora cavernosa and attempts to mimic the characteristics of an erect penis.

A penile prosthesis requires surgical implantation; placement of a penile prosthesis should be considered irreversible. The patient will not be able to use any other therapy to obtain an erection after a penile prosthesis is placed.

Modern prostheses consist of two major types:

Semi-rigid and inflatable

Erosion is more common with semi-rigid implants. Semi-rigid prostheses have been placed in patients to help improve the fit of chronic condom catheters. More manual dexterity is required for the inflatable prosthesis. Infection rate in primary implants is usually from 0 to 3%. Infection rates are higher in men with spinal cord injury, immunosuppression, steroid use, and diabetics with elevated glycosylated hemoglobin.

Diabetics with good glucose control probably have a similar infection rate as non-diabetics. Infection rates are higher in replacement or secondary penile implants and when multiple implants are placed at once (e.g. penile prosthesis and artificial urinary sphincter). Staphylococcus is the most common organism cultured.

The chance of prosthesis failure/malfunction requiring re-operation is approximately 5-10% at five years postoperatively. Satisfaction rates are high for both the patient (up to 89%) and the patient's partner (up to 70%). Those requiring additional operations were least satisfied.

What is the current role of penile prosthesis implantation?

With the introduction of sildenafil citrate [12], oral medication has become the first line therapy for erectile dysfunction. When systemic therapy fails or is contraindicated, second line treatments are considered, including vacuum devices, intraurethral medications, and intracavernosal injection therapy. Men who fail or reject second line therapies should be considered for penile prosthesis implantation provided that the erectile dysfunction is not primarily psychogenic.

Which various types of penile prostheses are available?

- Rod Prostheses
- Inflatable Prostheses
    - One-piece Inflatable devices
    - Two-piece Inflatable devices
    - Three-piece Inflatable devices

Rod Prostheses are paired solid devices implanted in the corpora that provide constant rigidity. Advantages include ease of implantation and freedom from mechanical faults. Disadvantages include a constantly rigid penis that resembles neither normal erection nor flaccidity, difficulties with concealment and an increased risk for device erosion [13].

Examples of rod prostheses are:

- Malleable 650 (AMS, USA)
- Mentor Malleable (Mentor, USA)
- Acu-Form (Mentor, USA)
- Dura-II (Timm Medical Technologies, USA)

One-piece Inflatable prostheses are not popular any longer. Examples of such prostheses include the Flexi-plate device manufactured by Surgitek, USA and Hydroflex and Dynaflex devices from American Medical Systems (AMS, USA).

Two-piece Inflatable devices consist of paired cylinders connected by tubing to a scrotal component. In the Ambicor prosthesis (AMS), the scrotal pump transfers fluid from the proximal portion of the cylinders to the distal portion resulting in rigidity without girth expansion. In the Mark-II device from Mentor, the scrotal component serves as both the pump and the reservoir.

Three-piece inflatable implants have paired cylinders, a small scrotal pump, and a large volume abdominal fluid reservoir. AMS makes three such prostheses. The 700CX device, introduced in 1987 produces controlled girth expansion and rigidity, the 700CXM, which has smaller cylinders and is now used primarily in men with fibrotic corpora. In 1990, they introduced the Ultrex Inflatable penile prostheses, which provides not only girth expansion and rigidity but also length expansion. This length expansion was however, associated with decreased cylinder longevity, and this issue has been addressed in the improved cylinders available since 1993 that possess a stronger middle layer. Mentor manufactures two such implants, the Alpha I, and the Alpha I Narrow Back for men with fibrotic corpora (post-priapism, post-infection).

Examples of penile prostheses:

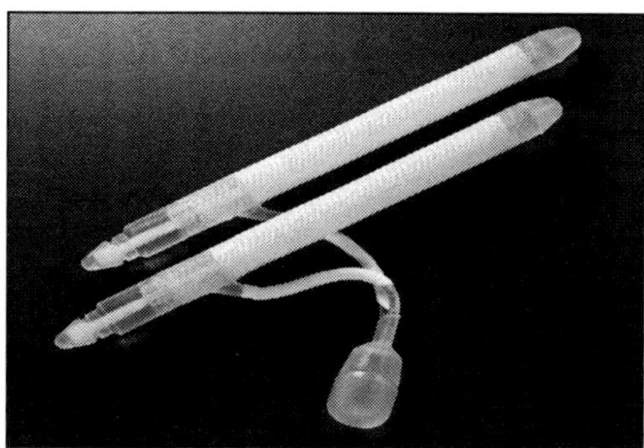

Ambicor Prostheses

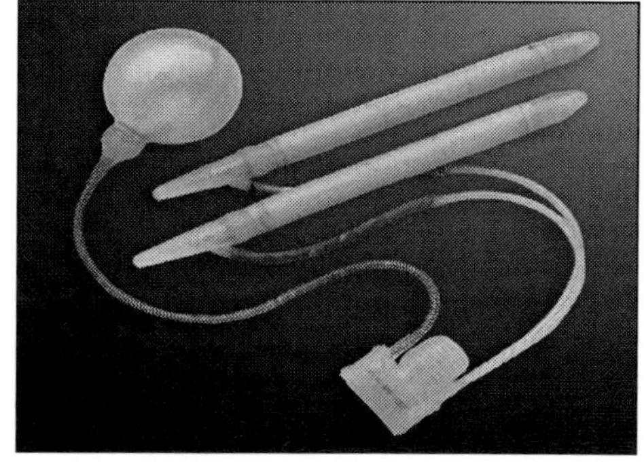

AMS 700 Penile Prosthesis with InhibiZone™

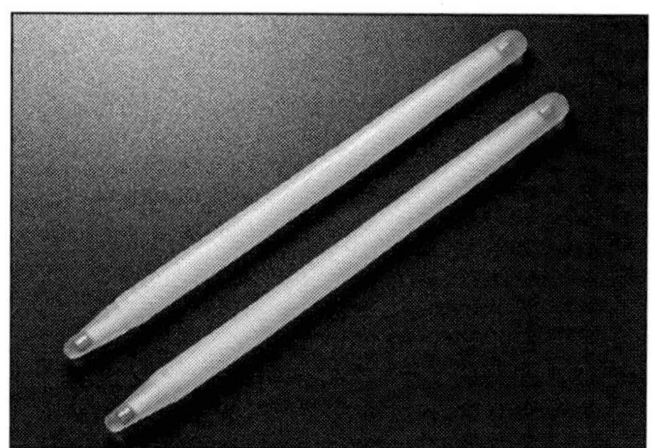

AMS 650 Semi-rigid

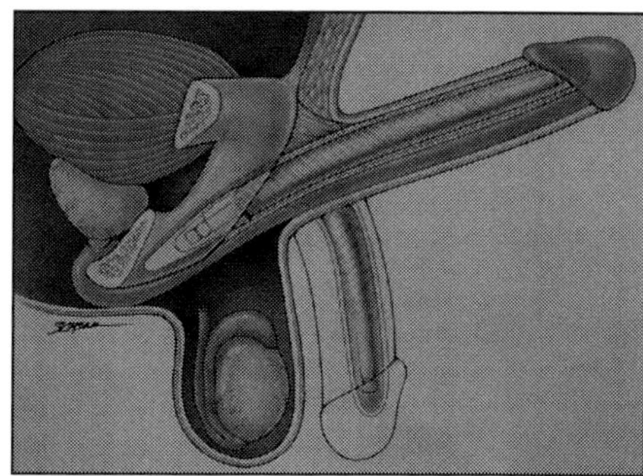

Ultrex device

How does one select which type of prosthesis to use in a given case?

The ideal penile prosthesis would allow a man to produce an erection and flaccidity of the penis that approximates, as closely as possible, the natural condition and also allows him to control when he has an erection. Only the three-piece inflatable device approaches this ideal with its large abdominal reservoir that transfers fluid into the expandable corporal cylinders. Currently, only the Ultrex device offers length expansion in addition to girth and rigidity and is the first choice for men presenting for first-time implantation.

The 700CX prosthesis is preferred for men with associated penile curvature (Peyronie's disease) because it has better straightening properties (13). Similarly for patients with a long penis, the CX device is preferred as it provides better rigidity at longer lengths. If the penis is small or the corpora fibrotic, the CXM device or the Alpha I Narrow Back may allow cylinder implantation with primary closure of the tunica albuginea. For men with previous erosion, the CX cylinders are preferred because avoidance of length expansion in these situations is desirable. For repeat cases if the penis is supple and stretchable, the Ultrex device can still be used successfully (13).

Can you discuss the salient points of surgical technique in the placement of three-piece penile prosthesis?

The preferred approach is made via a transverse scrotal incision as it offers unparalleled exposure of the corpora. The placement of the reservoir is by a blind technique. Great care is necessary during sizing of the prosthesis (especially the Ultrex device which is capable of length expansion) to avoid the S shaped cylinder deformity and premature wear or erosion. It is a good idea to pre-place sutures to close the corporotomy in order to avoid inadvertent puncture of the cylinders. The scrotal pump is placed in a scrotal subdartos pouch either in the midline or to one side. The reservoir is placed extraperitoneally in the retropubic space of Retzius under zero pressure and without any excess fluid in order to avoid autoinflation of the cylinders.

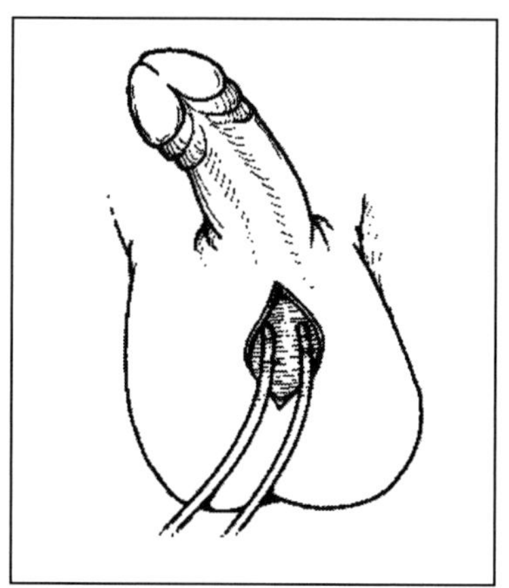

The incision for a penile implant may be for either a semi-rigid or an inflatable prosthesis. The illustrations show the inflatable form only. The principles and techniques for insertion are similar for both the semi-rigid and inflatable prosthesis although the equipment is different.

Figure 1.
An incision for a penile implant, which may be either semi-rigid or an inflatable prosthesis.

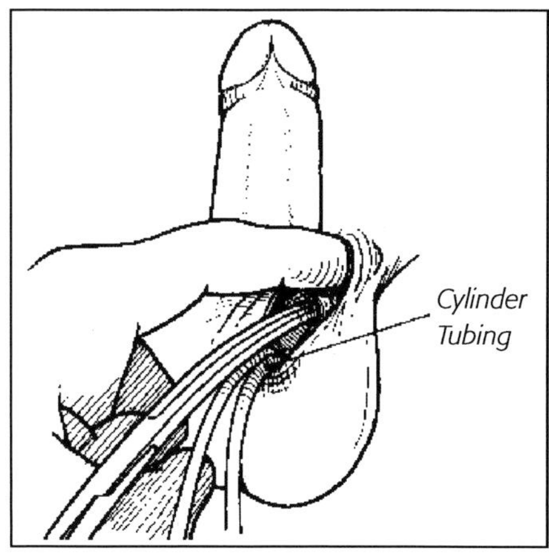

Figure 2.
After an incision has been made on the underside of the penis, the tissues on both sides of the urethra are expanded to allow placement of the implants.

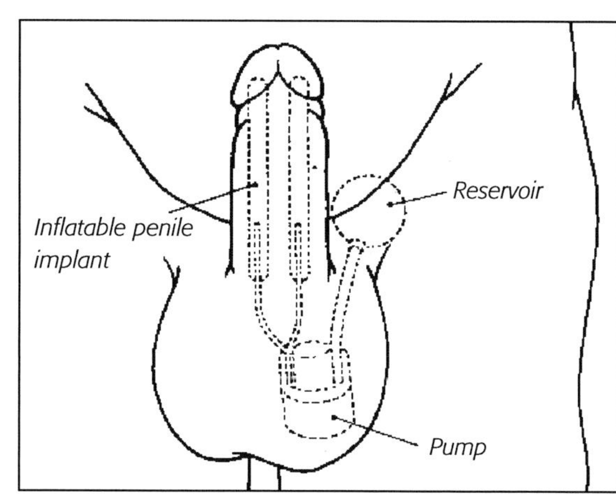

Figure 3.
Implants in place, the surgical incision is closed with absorbable sutures.

What is the treatment for periprosthetic infections?

The body reacts to silicone by forming a fibrous pseudocapsule around it. Infections in the space between this pseudocapsule and the silicone cylinders are called periprosthetic infections. Most are the result of the implant operation itself but some do occur much later due to blood borne spread of infection from a distant site. Jarow has reported a 1.8% infection rate in primary procedures and a 13.3% infection rate in secondary procedures[14]. Since these infections are associated with a biofilm of organisms on the prosthesis itself, they mandate complete removal of the implant for adequate control.

For many years, the standard procedure was to delay the new implant for six to 12 months, however, this leads to severe contraction of the fibrous scar tissue, shortening of the penis and great difficulty in corporal dilation and implantation at the later date. Current recommendations, therefore, are to use either salvage therapy or device removal with early re-implantation. Salvage therapy entails, in one operation, complete device removal, copious irrigation with a variety of solutions, re-draping, re-gloving, re-gowning, and re-implantation of a new prosthesis from a new instrument table. Mulcahy has reported 82% success with this salvage surgery[15]. An alternative is to re-implant within four to six weeks by which time the incision and drain sites of the prosthesis explantation operation have healed completely. Although fibrous tissue already exists by this time it has not contracted and the penile size is maintained. Dilation and re-implantation is thus technically easier.

ARTERIAL INSUFFICIENCY

Is there a place for penile revascularization?

Although the stepladder approach is the preferred strategy for arteriogenic ED, the allure of penile revascularization surgery is the potential to increase arterial blood flow sufficiently to the penis to restore normal physiologic erections, without the need of drugs or other adjuncts. Simply stated, penile revascularization involves direct arterial surgery to bypass an obstruction in the feeder arteries of the cavernosal arteries, with an aim to increase the arterial supply of the corpora cavernosa.

At the present time, revascularization is indicated in patients who meet all of the following criteria:

- Young men with traumatic arterial insufficiency or focal arterial defect on internal pudendal arteriogram
- No evidence of veno-occlusive dysfunction
- Have stopped smoking

The success rate in these patients is approximately 60%-70% at five years. Those with generalized atherosclerosis are not candidates for revascularization.

Revascularization is done by anastomosing the inferior epigastric artery to the dorsal penile artery. Revascularization has also been accomplished by anastomosing the inferior epigastric artery to the deep dorsal vein, but this often causes glans hyperemia, which is uncomfortable for the patient.

If the patient is not a candidate for revascularization, any of the therapies for assisted erection may be tried.

Surgery for veno-occlusive disorders:

For the rigid turgor of normal penile erection, increased arterial inflow has to be accompanied by adequate occlusion of the outflow veins of the penis. Failure of this veno-occlusive mechanism is an important cause of ED. It may result from:

- Presence or development of large venous channels draining the corpora cavernosa
- Degenerative changes or traumatic injury to the tunica resulting in inadequate compression of the subtunical and emissary veins
- Structural alterations in fibroelastic components of the corpora
- Insufficient trabecular smooth muscle relaxation, and
- Acquired venous shunts

What is the role of surgery for veno-occlusive disease?

Surgery for veno-occlusive dysfunction has largely fallen out of favor due to poor outcomes. In general, this is due to inappropriate patient selection for such surgery. The diagnosis of venous leak must be carefully distinguished from venous drainage which may occur in normal patients, particularly in the abnormal environment of a radiology suite during invasive testing! Appearance of rapidly filling venous channels on cavernosometry that follow normal anatomical routes does not confirm veno-occlusive dysfunction. There are certain features observed on color Doppler ultrasound (Vmax >25cm/sec; Vmin >5 cm/sec) and dynamic cavernosometry (maintenance flow rate > 15-20 ml/min), which can be used to reach this diagnosis.

Management of patients in whom veno-occlusive function is diagnosed should again begin with less invasive treatment options, as pharmacotherapy may succeed for some and vacuum devices may also be appropriate. Venous ligation surgery results in only approximately 30% improvement in reported series, most of which have follow up of less than 24 months. Penile revascularization and embolization for venous problems carry similarly unattractive results, and ultimately implantation of a prosthesis may be the preferred surgical option.

A suggested algorithm for the stepwise management of ED is as follows [11]:

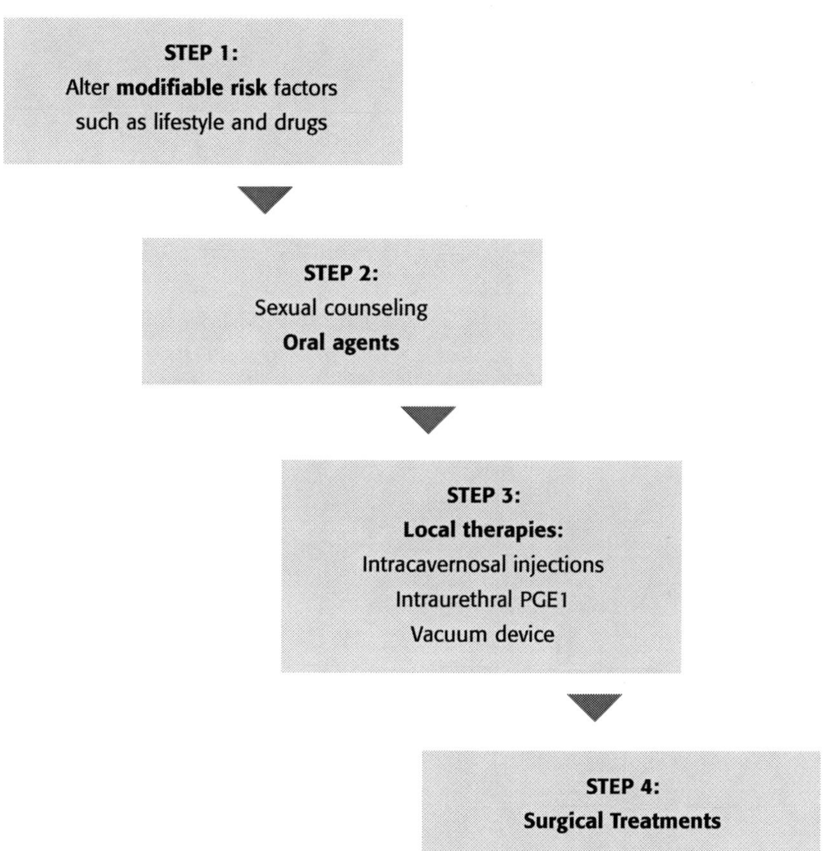

CHAPTER EIGHT

PEYRONIE'S DISEASE

What is Peyronies' disease and how do you treat it?

Peyronie's disease ('induratio penis plastica') is characterized by the formation of an inelastic scar (plaque) in the tunica albuginea of the corpora cavernosa, which often results in penile curvature. It may be associated with Dupuytren's contracture of the palmar fascia, Ledderhose's disease of the plantar fascia, and tympanosclerosis of the eardrum [(1)].

The cause of Peyronie's disease is not well understood; one possible cause is trauma during vigorous sexual activity [(2)].

The plaque remodels over the course of a year or so. After this time, the plaque becomes stable and may even resolve; plaque calcification indicates that the plaque has finished remodeling [(3)]. Pain may occur in up to 66% of men, especially in the acute phase of remodeling when the inflammatory response is peaking.

Treatment

During the acute phase, treatment is aimed at controlling inflammation, relieving pain, and preventing progression of the plaque.

Various regimens using non-surgical agents are outlined below:

- Vitamin E 1000-1500 IU q day [4].
- Amino benzoate potassium (Potaba® Envules) 3 g orally four times daily. It usually takes at least two to three months of therapy before effects can be observed. The drug may improve both pain and penile deformation [5].
- Colchicine 0.6 mg orally three times daily [6].
- Non steroidal anti-inflammatory drugs.
- Other possible therapies include, intralesional steroid injections, oral tamoxifen, and shock wave therapy.

None of the above medical therapies stands scrutiny in terms of controlled trial data. It would not be unreasonable to suggest that use of any of the above medical regimens or shock wave lithotripsy should be confined to the setting of a carefully designed clinical trial.

After the acute phase, treatment is based on patient preference and degree of sexual dysfunction. If the patient and partner are satisfied with their sexual function, no therapy is required. If they are not satisfied, then surgical options are available. Surgical therapy is only performed if the plaque has finished maturation otherwise the patient may have plaque progression post surgery [7].

Surgical options :

- Plication; patients are counseled regarding the possible loss of erect penile length prior to surgery.
- Plaque incision and grafting (vein or other biologic matrix); this is more suitable for the patient with severe deformity (>30 degrees) and possibly for those with shorter penile length. Theoretically, there is a reduced likelihood of shortening, but this is not borne out in all published series.
- If the patient has Peyronie's disease and erectile dysfunction with poor response to less invasive erection therapies, then placement of a penile prosthesis may be performed.

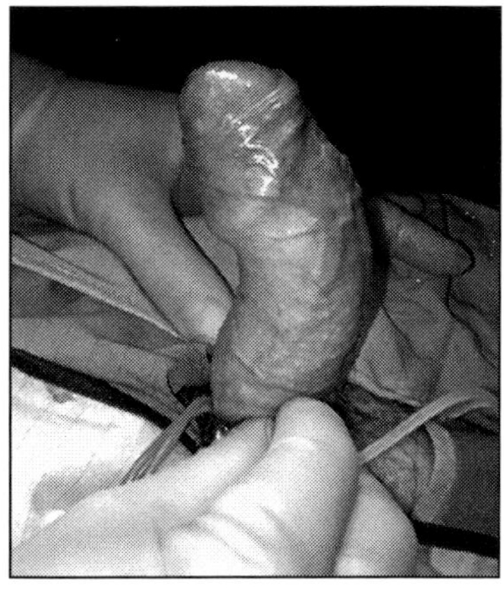

Preoperative artificial erection showing marked angulation

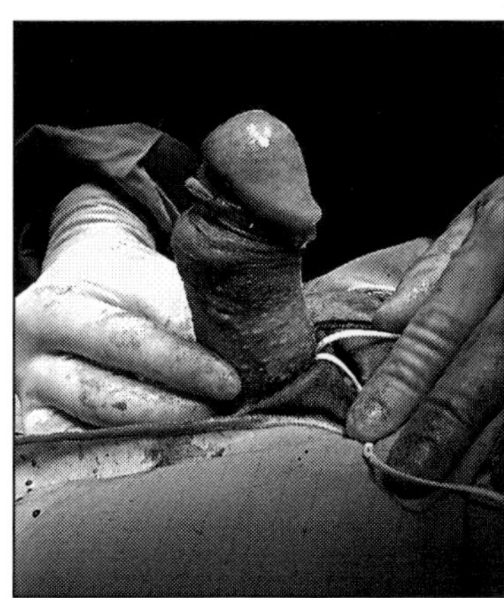

Postoperative picture showing straightening out of the angulation

CHAPTER NINE

PREMATURE EJACULATION

What exactly is premature ejaculation?

There is no consensus on the definition of premature ejaculation. A working definition is: 'male ejaculation that occurs too early for female partner satisfaction in at least 50% of attempts'.

The incidence of this problem is high, approximately 35% [1], and it is the most common form of male sexual dysfunction. This raises the obvious question of whether the condition is truly organic in nature or merely consists of normal sexual function associated with abnormal expectations [2].

The etiology of premature ejaculation may include [3]:

- Congenital
- Psychological/Behavioral (the commonest cause)
- Chemical substances (e.g. opioid withdrawal)

Treatment

Treatment options include systemic therapy, topical therapy and behavioral/psychological therapies. The goal of therapy is to increase patient control over the ejaculation process by decreasing penile sensitivity and adjusting the behavioral response [2].

SYSTEMIC MEDICAL THERAPY

Clomipramine

This is a tricyclic antidepressant that inhibits the reuptake of serotonin. Clomipramine 25 mg orally once daily is the initial dose. The dose may be increased to 50 mg and the dosing frequency may be decreased to every other day or less depending on side effects. Side effects include dry mouth, constipation, sleep disturbances, nausea, fatigue, hot flashes, and seizures.

Clomipramine and monoamine oxidase inhibitors (MAOI) are not to be used in combination. Using clomipramine with MAOI's can cause fatal reactions. The patient should be off MAOI's for at least five weeks before starting clomipramine. Clomipramine can lower the seizure threshold; therefore, clomipramine should be avoided in patients with a history of seizures or at risk for seizures (e.g. brain lesions, brain damage, alcoholism, or use of other drugs that lower seizure threshold).

Selective serotonin reuptake inhibitors (SSRI's)

SSRI's are antidepressants and are a logical choice for treatment of premature ejaculation as they induce an ejaculation. They have been studied in placebo-controlled, randomized, and blinded trials and have shown efficacy in prolonging time to ejaculation.

Special precautions: Use of SSRI's with monoamine oxidase inhibitors may cause fatal reactions; usage of both drugs together is contraindicated.

Side effects
Nausea, diarrhea, anorexia, tremor, nervousness, dizziness, sleep disturbances, increased sweating, and dry mouth.

Each of the following SSRI's may be tried:

- Sertraline 50 mg orally once daily is the initial dose. At least one week must pass before each increase in the dose. Maximum dose is 200 mg orally once daily.
- Fluoxetine 20 mg orally once daily is the initial dose. After several weeks, the dose may be increased to 20 mg po BID if needed.
- Paroxetine 20 mg orally once daily is the initial dose. At least one week must pass before each increase in the dose. The dose may be increased in 10 mg/day increments up to a maximum of 50 mg/day as needed.

Topical Therapy

Topical anesthetics such as 2% lidocaine jelly, have been used anecdotally to decrease penile sensitivity and prolong ejaculatory latency. A recent trial has reported an 80% success with the topical use of EMLA (Eutectic Mixture of Local Anesthetics) cream 30 minutes prior to intercourse [4]. A herbal preparation called SS-cream has also been demonstrated to increase ejaculatory latency by tenfold without anesthetic action on the female tract [2].

Behavioral Therapy

For durable success in the treatment of PME, systemic or local therapies must be combined with behavioral modification. Cooperation of the partner is of paramount importance. Such therapy seeks to provide enhanced patient control and satisfaction from sexual stimulation. The patient and the partner together undergo several weeks of sex therapy in which they learn relaxation techniques and acquire skills to perform prolonged (15 minutes) self or partner-performed sexual stimulation without the demand for ejaculation. Subsequently patients are instructed in methods of passive coitus without thrusting and eventually coitus with pelvic thrusting [2].

CHAPTER TEN

PRIAPISM

What is priapism?

History: The word priapism has origins in Greek mythology. Priapus, the God of fertility and luck, was born in Asia Minor, most likely the son of Aphrodite. Priapus is believed to have a deformed body with a markedly enhanced phallus. Tripe is credited with the first medical report of priapism in 1841[1].

Definition: Priapism is a pathologic condition of a penile erection that persists beyond or is unrelated to sexual stimulation. Except in cases of nonischemic type, priapism is often accompanied by pain and tenderness.

Hemodynamically, priapism can be separated into two distinct types:

- Low flow (ischemic) priapism (Type I priapism)
- High flow (non-ischemic) priapism (Type 2 priapism)

Etiology: Traditionally, priapism has been classified as primary/idiopathic, wherein there is no obvious predisposing cause, and secondary, due to diseases such as leukemia, sickle cell disease, penile trauma, drug abuse, or intracavernosal injection therapy for impotence [2]. It can also present as acute, intermittent (recurring\stuttering), or chronic (usually in the high-flow type) [3].

How does this condition present?

Clinical presentation will vary but most patients present with a history of several hours of painful erection. Typically, priapism affects only the corpora cavernosa, in rare cases the corpus spongiosum is also involved [4]. The ventral surface of the erect penis is flat since the bulge of the erect spongiosum, which surrounds the urethra in a normal erection, is missing. Tenderness to palpation is variable, but increases with time. Ischemic priapism is a failure of the detumescence mechanism from many causes, among which are excessive release of neurotransmitters, blockage of draining venules, paralysis of intrinsic detumescence mechanism, and prolonged relaxation of the intracavernous smooth muscles.

This has an important bearing on the potential to vascular thrombosis accompanied by fibrosis of the erectile tissue and can lead to impotence in as high as 50% of patients. However, all patients will regain their previous potency if the priapism is aborted within 12 to 24 hours by medical therapy [5]. Priapism is a urological emergency and must be treated as such.

How is acute priapism managed?

A 21 gauge butterfly needle is inserted into either corpora cavernosa and blood aspirated. This is usually quite dark and an initial sample is sent for blood gas determination to document the degree of ischemia. Ten to twenty ml of blood is aspirated at a time and replaced with an equal amount of normal saline. Ideally, this should be repeated until no dusky colored blood remains and thereafter 5 ml of diluted phenylephrine is injected into the corpora; this diluted phenylephrine is prepared by taking 1 ml of a solution containing 10 mg of the drug and diluting it to 100 ml with normal saline. The process is repeated at 10-minute intervals until the erection subsides [(5)]. Patients receiving phenylephrine should be monitored (blood pressure and pulse) because tachycardia, tachyarrythmia, and hypertension may result when the priapism resolves and the phenylephrine is released into the systemic circulation.

Treatment of secondary priapism would depend on the specific cause. Patients with sickle-cell disease have benefited from hydration, oxygenation and alkalinization. Super-transfusion and erythropheresis should be used as second-line therapy. Patients with leukemia should receive prompt chemotherapy if possible [(6)]. Treatment of high flow non-ischemic priapism consequent to trauma is usually established by color duplex ultrasonography. This is subsequently treated by internal pudendal arteriography and selective embolization of the artery feeding the shunt [(7)].

If non-operative treatment of this type of priapism fails, a shunting procedure is indicated. A corporo-glandular shunt is the first reasonable approach. If this does not work, a corporo-spongiosal shunt is performed [8].

What are the different types of shunts?

Corporo-glandular (CG) shunts:

- **Winter shunt:** a Tru-cut biopsy needle is inserted into the glans penis to excise multiple cores between the distal corpora cavernosa and the glans. If this does not work, an open surgical shunt is required.
- **Ebbehoj shunt:** a stab incision is made in the glans, and the blade is rotated to create a communication between the corpora cavernosa and the glans.
- **Al-Ghorab Shunt:** a 2 cm transverse incision is made in the dorsal glans penis 1 cm distal to the coronal sulcus. The distal portion of tunica albuginea is excised from each corpora.

Corporo-spongiosal (CS) shunts:

- **Quackel's Shunt:** Through a perineal or penile shaft incision, the corpus spongiosum and corpus cavernosum are incised and anastomosed on one side. The more proximal the shunt, the less likely a urethral fistula will occur because the thickness of the spongiosum covering the urethra is greater.

- **Corporo-saphenous shunt (Grayhack shunt):** the saphenous vein is mobilized and anastomosed to the corpus cavernosum at the base of the penis.

A suggested algorithm for the treatment of priapism is as follows [9]:

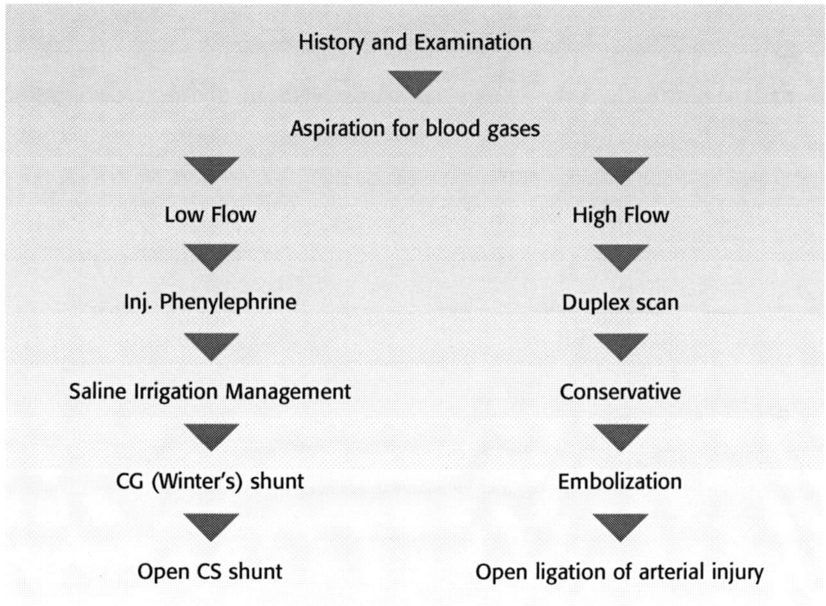

What is the role of penile implants in priapism?

Many cases of low flow priapism will unfortunately present late. It is probably still appropriate to follow the suggested treatment algorithm, even as far as performing a shunt procedure, but ultimately a significant number will have resultant ED necessitating implantation of a prosthesis.

Late implantation (beyond two weeks) may prove very difficult due to the presence of severe fibrosis, and these patients comprise a special group requiring the presence of particular surgical expertise. Recently, Ralph [10] et al have reported on a series employing early penile prosthesis implantation with encouraging results. This group employs adjunctive use of frozen section penile biopsy to confirm smooth muscle necrosis and their work deserves careful attention.

CHAPTER ELEVEN

A LOOK TO THE FUTURE

It would have been hard to imagine 10 years ago that we would now be successfully treating ED with tablets. This field has come a long way since the launch of sildenafil citrate and it seems likely given the speed of advance up until now, that further developments are on the horizon.

Currently, the pharmaceutical producers of ED drugs are aggressively marketing their products' individual characteristics, suggesting particular benefits associated with different pharmacological properties. This may be an overly simplistic way of alluding to differences in the efficacy of the PDE5 inhibitors, but in the absence of direct comparative data, we must continue to rely on real life experience with our use of these products.

We now have a number of PDE5s available and this gives our patients the opportunity to "road test" each, to assess personal preference, which may well be the result of individual idiosyncrasies rather than pharmacology. Newer PDE5 inhibitors will appear, and while we will watch with interest their evolution into the treatment armamentarium, it seems likely that we will continue to rely on the presently available agents for some time yet. The other, currently available drug therapies, have a limited, but continuing use in selected patients.

This chapter will deal with some of the potentially exciting developments in laboratory and clinical research in the field of erectile dysfunction, with particular reference to potential therapeutic agents that may have a role in the coming years.

What are the biochemical processes involved in erection?

Nitric oxide (NO) is the principal mediator of erection, and its role has been previously outlined in an earlier section of this book. We are aware that NO is derived both from cavernous nerve endings and from endothelial cells, and that depletion of this transmitter substance is observed in certain forms of ED. Successful therapy has, not surprisingly therefore centered around compounds like the PDE5 inhibitors, which effectively increase the available NO and its second messenger agents (cGMP/ G kinase; cAMP/ A kinase). It may also be theoretically possible to introduce agents, which supplement NO levels in ED patients where the basal level in the disease process is reduced. In a rabbit model, a nitric oxide releasing PDE5 inhibitor (NCX-911) showed promising results.

What we have been less clear on however, are the processes, which regulate flaccidity or maintain erection. Studies have now shown that a variety of vasoactive substances appear to play regulatory roles in the penis in both disease and health [2].

Noradrenalin (NA) and endothelin-1 (ET-1) are the most potent of these, and as vasoconstrictors, elicit an increase in intracellular calcium, resulting in smooth muscle contraction. There is "upstream" regulation of these vasoconstrictors by the Rho A/ Rho kinase system, a calcium-sensitizing pathway involved in the regulation of the cellular events of smooth muscle contraction [3]. Inhibition of smooth muscle activity would, in theory, promote smooth muscle relaxation and hence erection. Animal studies of Rho kinase inhibition with Y-27632 have shown it to produce erection independent of NO, but remains at a relatively early pre-clinical stage of development [4].

Other chemicals, such as Growth Hormone (GH) and Angiotensin Converting Enzyme (ACE) have also been demonstrated to have a role in the control of tumescence, but their value as therapeutic targets remain to be exploited further.

What is the place of centrally acting drugs in current ED management?

The Dopamine agonist apomorphine has been in clinical use widely for a number of years. Results of trial data have not been mirrored in real life clinical practice, where some men with mild or short duration ED benefit. Outcomes are not favorable when compared to PDE5 inhibitors, and its practical role is limited [5,6]. There may be a place for this drug in the management of both male and female libido disorders, but study data from intranasal administration and second generation dopamine agonists are awaited.

The other centrally acting group of compounds of interest are melanocortin receptor agonists. Melanocortin receptors (Type IV) appear to be involved in the erectile process and injection of a study compound (PT-141) has shown a degree of clinical efficacy compared to placebo. As with apomorphine, nausea is a frequently reported problem, but improvements in sexual desire have also been reported [(7)].

Is there still a role for PGE1 (Alprostadil) in the PDE5 era?

Clearly, much of the impetus behind the development of oral agents to treat ED was the lack of acceptability of intracavernosal PGE1 injection. While almost universally effective in producing erection, self-injection results in poor long term patient acceptance and compliance [(8)]. There is no evidence to state that other injected agents fare better. MUSE, developed in 1997 as a more palatable alternative to injection, has not been particularly effective as a first line agent in ED due to limited efficacy.

Topical application is for some an attractive alternative however, and may be appropriate in those for whom PDE5 therapy is contraindicated, or for those whose treatment choice is influenced by the wish to minimize risk of potential side effects. As such, trials of topically applied alprostadil with an absorption enhancing agent (Topiglan), have been carried out in both a feline model and ED patients. In the animal studies, a dose-dependent increase in intracavernosal pressures was observed to a point where a 1%

concentration of the substance topically was equivalent to an effective injected dose [9]. In patients however, while a significant difference over placebo was demonstrated, it was clear that further stimulation by audiovisual or tactile means, improved the erection further. This suggested a facilitatory rather than initiating role for topical PGE110.

What are the latest developments in gene therapy for ED?

The perceived role of gene therapies in medicine has been that of high risk, high cost technology to treat potentially life-threatening disorders with a easily identifiable genetic basis. Therefore, it requires a significant shift in our thinking to consider this as a potential avenue for the progress in ED management.

However, it is evident from much we have said previously, that the physiology of erection can be manipulated by targeting clearly identified biochemical pathways. If this could be achieved, there might be a viable alternative for those in whom conventional ED therapies are not effective, or who wish a more natural resolution to their sexual difficulties without the planning that conventional treatment entails.

As nitric oxide is the prime mediator of erection, it is natural that the NO/nitric oxide synthase (NOS) pathway has been the target for much of the laboratory based gene therapy experiments to date. So far, all the isoforms of NOS have been targeted in rodent models. Success has been achieved in terms of physiological effect (measured increase in intracavernosal pressure), but the major limitation has been short duration of gene expression, and hence longevity of effect [11,12,13].

A significant advance has been made by one New York based group who have targeted the hSlo gene via transfer of a naked DNA plasmid vector. The gene product in question is the maxi-K ion channel, a potassium channel closely associated with calcium flux and control of corporal smooth muscle tone.

Overexpression of the hslo gene results in enhancement of smooth muscle responsiveness. In a rodent model, effect was seen for up to six months in aged rats and four months in diabetic rats [14]. This work has now been carried forward into phase I clinical trials [15].

Other research in this area using gene therapy with calcitonin gene related peptide, VEGF and brain derived neurotrophic factor are also ongoing, and will no doubt report in the future.

REFERENCES

Introduction References

1. Impotence. In NIH consensus statement online 1992: 1-31.
2. Shah J. Erectile dysfunction through the ages. BJU Int, 2002; 90: 433-441.
3. Bhishagratna KK. The Sushruta Samhita. An English translation based on the original Sanskrit text, 2nd ed. Varanasi, India: Chowkhamba Sanskrit Series Office, 1963.
4. Levey M. The medicinal formulary of Aqrabadhin of Al-Kindhi. Madison: University of Wisconsin Press, 1966.
5. Ebrey P. Chinese civilization: A sourcebook. 2nd ed. New York: Free Press, 1993.
6. Li CL. A brief outline of Chinese medical history with particular reference to acupuncture. Perspect Biol Med, 1974; 18: 132-143.
7. Smith GE. Papyrus Ebers. English translation. Chicago: Ares Publishers, 1974.
8. Cotton N. Castrating witches. Impotence and magic in the Merry Wives of Windsor. Shakespeare, W. 1987; 3: 320-326.
9. Darmon P. Damning the innocent: A history of the persecution of the impotent in pre-revolutionary France. London: Hogarth Press, 1985.
10. Haller JS. Spermatic economy. A 19th century view of male impotence. Southern Med J 1989; 82: 1010-6.
11. Belt E. Leonardo the Florentine (1452-1519). Invest Urol 1965; 3: 99-106.
12. Hansen B. New images of a new medicine: Visual evidence for the widespread popularity of therapeutic discoveries in America after 1885. Bull Hist Med 1999; 73: 629-78.

13. Macht T, Teagarden E. Rejuvenation experiments with vas ligation in rats. J Urol 1923; 10: 407-11.

14. Taberner PV. Aphrodisiacs – the science and the myth. Philadelphia: The University of Pennsylvania Press, 1985.

15. Gee WF. The history of surgical treatment of impotence. Urology 1975; 5: 401-5.

16. Borgoras NA. Uber die volle plastiche weiderherstellung eines rum koitus fahigen penis (peniplastica totalis). Zentralbl Chir 1936; 63: 1271.

17. Bergman RT, Howard AH, Barnes RW. Plastic reconstruction of the penis. J Urol 1948; 59: 1174.

18. Goodwin WE, Scott WW. Phalloplasty. J Urol 1952; 68: 903

19. Beheri GE. Surgical treatment of impotence. Plast Reconst Surg 1966; 38: 92.

20. Pearman RO. Treatment of organic impotence by implantation of a penile prosthesis. J Urol 1967; 97: 716-9.

21. Small MP, Carrion HM, Gordon JA. Small-Carrion penile prosthesis: new implant for management of impotence. Urology 1975; 5: 479.

22. Finney RP. New hinged silicone penile implant. J Urol 1977; 118: 585.

23. Scott FB, Bradley WE, Timm GW. Management of erectile impotence: use of implantable inflatable prosthesis. Urology 1973; 2: 80.

24. Virag R, Virag H. Trial of intracavernous papaverine in the treatment of impotence: therapeutic prospects. J Mal Vasc 1983; 8: 293-5.

Chapter 1 References

1. Lewis RW. Epidemiology of erectile dysfunction. The Urologic Clinics of North America, 2001; 28(2): 209-216.

2. Spector IP, Carey MP. Incidence and the prevalence of the sexual dysfunctions: A critical review of the empirical literature. Arch sex Behav 1990; 19: 389.

3. Laumann EO, Gagnon JH, Michael RT, et al. The social organization of sexuality. Sexual practices in the United States. Chicago, University of Chicago Press, 1994.

4. Laumann EO, Paik A, Rosen R. Sexual dysfunction in the United States: Prevalence and predictors. JAMA, 1999; 21: 537.

5. Feldman HA, Goldstein I, Hatzichristou DG, Krane RJ, McKinlay JB. Impotence and its medical and psychological correlates: results of the Massachusetts Male Aging Study. J Urol.1994; 151: 54-61.

6. Spector KR, Boyle M. The prevalence and perceived etiology of male sexual problems:a non-clinical sample. Br J Med Psychol 1996; 59: 351.

7. Malmsten UGH, Milson I, Molander U, et al. Urinary incontinence and lower urinary tract symptoms: An epidemiological study of men aged 45 to 99 years. J Urol 1997; 158: 1733.

8. Fugl-Meyer AR, Sjogren Fugl-Meyer K. Sexual disabilities, problems and satisfaction in 18-74 year old Swedes. Scand J Sexol 1999; 2: 79.

9. Bejin A. Epidemiologie d'ejaculation premature et de son cumul avec la dysfunction erectile. Andrologie, 1999; 9: 211.

10. Chew KK, Earle CM, Stuckey BGA, et al. Erectile dysfunction in general medical practice: Prevalence and clinical correlates. Int J Impotence Res 2000; 12: 41.

11. Rosen, R.C., Fisher, W.A., Eardley, I. et al. The multinational Men's Attitudes to Life Events and Sexuality (MALES) study: 1. Prevalence of erectile dysfunction and related health concerns in the general population. Curr Med Res Op 2004; 20(5): 603-17.

12. Aytac, I.A., McKinlay, J.B., Krane, R.J. The likely world-wide increase in erectile dysfunction between 1995 and 2025 and some possible policy consequences. BJU Int 1999; 84: 50-6.

Chapter 2 References

1. Andersson, K.E. Erectile physiological and pathophysiological pathways involved in erectile dysfunction. J Urol, 170: S6-14, 2003.

2. Lue, T.F. Erectile dysfunction. N Engl J Med, 342: 1802-1813.

Chapter 7 References

1. Rosen RC, Capelleri JC, Smith MD, et al. Development and evaluation of an abridged, 5-item version of the International Index of Erectile Function (IIEF-5) as a diagnostic tool for erectile dysfunction. Int J Impot Res 1999; 11: 319.

2. Meuleman EJ, Broderick GA, Tan HM, et al. Clinical evaluation and the doctor-patient dialogue. In Jardin A, Wagner G, Khoury S, et al (eds.): Erectile Dysfunction: First International Consultation on Erectile Dysfunction. July 1-3, Paris, 1999, Plymouth, United Kingdom. Health Publication Ltd, 2000, pp 117-38.

3. Feldman HA, Goldstein I, Hatzichristou DG, Krane RJ, McKinlay JB. Impotence and its medical and psychological correlates: results of the Massachusetts Male Aging Study. J Urol.1994; 151: 54-61.

4. Ignarro LJ, Bush PA, Buga GM, et al. Nitric oxide and cyclic GMP formation upon electrical field stimulation cause relaxation of corpus cavernosum smooth muscle. Biochem Biophys Res Comm 1990; 170: 843-50.

5. Lizza EF, Rosen RC. Definition and classification of erectile dysfunction: Report of the nomenclature committee of the International Society of Impotence Research. Int J Impot Res 1999; 11: 141-43.

6. Carrier S, Brock G, Kour NW, Lue TF: Pathophysiology of erectile dysfunction. Urology 1993; 42: 468-81.

7. Krane RJ, Goldstein I, saenz de Tejada I. Impotence. N Engl J Med. 1989; 321: 1648-1659 abridged, 5-item version of the International Index of Erectile Function (IIEF-5) as a diagnostic tool for erectile dysfunction. Int J Impot Res 1999; 11: 319.

8. Davis-Joseph B, Tiefer L, Melman A: Accuracy of the initial history and physical examination to establish etiology of erectile dysfunction. Urology 1995; 45: 498-502.

9. Korenman SG. Clinical review 71: Advances in the understanding and management of erectile dysfunction. J Clin Endocrinol Metab.1995; 80: 985-88.

10. Broderick GA, Lue TF. Evaluation and nonsurgical management of Erectile dysfunction and priapism. Campbell's Urology, eighth edition. Walsh PC, Retik AB, Vaughan ED Jr and Wein AJ (eds.). Philadelphia: W. B. Saunders Company, 2002, pp 1619-71.

11. Jardin A, Wagner G, Khoury S. Recommendations of the 1st International Consultation on Erectile Dysfunction. In Jardin A, Wagner G, Khoury S, Giuliano F, Padma-Nathan H, Rosen R eds, Erectile Dysfunction. Plymouth UK: Health Publication Ltd, 2000: 709-26.

12. Goldstein I, Lue TF, Padma-Nathan H, et al. Oral sildenafil in the treatment of erectile dysfunction. Sildenafil study group. N Engl J Med, 338: 1397, 1998.

13. Montague DK, Angermeier KW. Penile prosthesis implantation. Urol Clin North Am, 2001; 28(2): 355-361.

14. Jarow JP. Risk factors for penile prosthetic infection. J Urol 1996; 156: 402.

15. Mulcahy JJ. Long-term experience with salvage of infected penile implants. J J Urol 2000; 163: 481.

Chapter 8 References

1. Ralph DJ, Schwartz G, Moore W et al. The genetic and bacteriological aspects of Peyronie's disease. J Urol 1997; 157: 291-94.
2. Somers KD, Dawson DM. Fibrin deposition in Peyronie's disease plaque. J Urol 1997; 157: 311-15.
3. Gelbard MK, Dorsey F, James K. The natural history of Peyronie's disease. J Urol 1990; 144: 1376-79.
4. Scardino PL, Scott WW. The use of tocopherols in the treatment of Peyronie's disease. Ann N Y Acad Sci 1949; 52: 390.
5. Zarafonetis CJD, Horrax TM. Treatment of Peyronie's disease with potassium para-aminobenzoate (Potaba), J Urol 1953; 81: 770-72.
6. Akkus E, Carrier S, Rehman J, et al. Is iarrhea less effective in Peyronie's disease? A pilot study. Urology 1994; 44: 291-95.
7. Lewis RW, Jordan GH. Surgery for erectile dysfunction. Campbell's Urology, eighth edition. Walsh PC, Retik AB, Vaughan ED Jr and Wein AJ. Philadelphia: W. B. Saunders Company, 2002, pp 1619-71.

Chapter 9 References

1. Read S, King M, Watson J. Sexual dysfunction in primary medical care: prevalence, characteristics and detection by the general practitioner. J Public Health Med 1997; 19: 387.
2. Master VA, Turek PJ. Ejaculatory physiology and dysfunction. Urol Clin North Am 2001; 28(2): 363-375.
3. Seftel, A. D. and Althof, S. E.: Premature ejaculation. W. J. G. Hellstrom (ed.), Male Infertility and Sexual Dysfunction. New York: Springer-Verlag New York, Inc., 1997, pp 356-361.

4. Berkovitch M, Keresteci AG, Koren G. Efficacy of prilocaine-lidocaine cream in the treatment of premature ejaculation. J Urol 1995; 154: 1360.

Chapter 10 References

1. Tripe JW. Case of continued priapism. Lancet 1845; 2: 8.

2. Pohl J, Pott B, Kleinhans G. Priapism: A three-phase concept of management according to etiology and prognosis. Br J Urol 1986; 58: 113.

3. Hashmat AI, Rehman J. Priapism. In Hashmat AI, Das S (eds.): The Penis. Philadelphia, Lea and Febiger, 1993, pp 219-43.

4. Shrapsteen JR, Powars D, Johnson C et al. Multisystem damage associated with tricorporal priapism in sickle cell disease. Am J Med 1993; 94: 289-95.

5. Kulmala RV, Tammela TL. Effects of priapism lasting 24 hours or longer caused by intracavernosal injection of vasoactive drugs. Int J Impot Res 1995; 7: 131-36.

6. Lue TF, Hellstorm WJ, McAninch JW, Tanagho EA. Priapism: A refined approach to diagnosis and treatment. J Urol 1986; 136: 104-8.

7. Brock G, Breza J, Lue TF, Tanagho EA. High flow priapism: A spectrum of disease. J Urol 1993; 150: 968-71.

8. Padma-Nathan H. Surgical management of priapism. Urol Clin North Am 1993; 1: 109-15

9. Pautler SE, Brock GB. Priapism: From Priapus to the present time. Urol Clin North Am, 2001; 28(2): 391-403.

10. The management of low-flow priapism with the immediate insertion of a penile prosthesis' Rees RW, Kalsi J, Minhas S, Peters J, Kell P, Ralph DJ BJU Int. 2002 Dec;90(9):893-7.

A TO Z INDEX

C

D

F

G

H

I

Q

R

S

T

NOTES